I0775335

LOW CARB 2024

LOW CARB 2024

Smart Snacking For Weight Loss Unveiling the Low Carb Delights - No Sugar, Quest Bars, and More

Deborah L Brooks

Copyright © [2023] by Deborah L Brooks

All rights reserved. No part of this book may be reproduced, stored, or transmitted in any form or by any means, electronic or mechanical, including photocopying, recording, or by any information storage and retrieval system, without the written permission of the author.

Disclaimer

The information provided in "Weight Maintenance 40+ Time Saver" is intended for general informational purposes only. The author, Deborah L Brooks and the publisher make no representations or warranties of any kind, express or implied, about the completeness, accuracy, reliability, suitability, or availability concerning the content contained within.

This book is not intended to provide medical, legal, or professional advice. Readers are encouraged to consult with relevant professionals for advice tailored to their specific situations. The author and publisher disclaim any liability for any loss or damage incurred as a result of the use of the information presented in this book.

While every effort has been made to ensure that the information in this book is accurate and up-to-date, the rapidly changing nature of certain fields may render some information obsolete. The author and publisher accept no responsibility for any consequences arising from the use of outdated information.

LOW CARB 2024

By reading this book, you agree that the author and publisher are not responsible for the success or failure of your personal or professional decisions related to the information presented herein.

About The Author

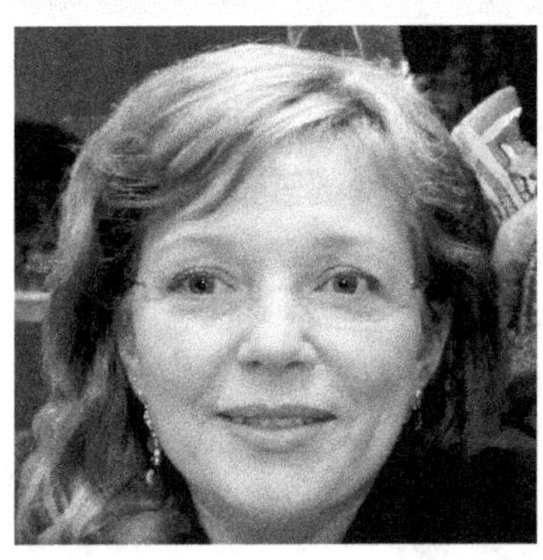

Hello, beautiful spirit! My name is Deborah L Brooks and I am the driving force behind "Low Carb 2024 ." Settle in, and allow me to tell you a little bit more about the person who writesZerothese pages.

I'm not your average writer; instead, I'm your go-to person for wellness and your co-conspirator while you manage your busy 40s. Think of me as the friend who gets really thrilled about spilling the beans about life's tiny secrets, particularly about embracing joy and health in this amazing decade.

Let's explore my planet now. I firmly think that eating should be quite enjoyable in addition to providing nourishment. I give away the beans (or maybe quinoa) on these pages about how to turn every meal into a celebration that delves into the worlds of flavor and mindfulness in addition to calories.

But there's more to it than just culinary misadventures. It's about the 1940s, a misinterpreted decade of existence. I want to be your confidante more than I want to be an author. This book is a dialogue, not a monologue. Get in touch with me via my website and social media accounts, tell me about yourself, pose inquiries, or just give me a virtual high five.

Now let's set off on this adventure together. I'm not simply a writer; one delectable recipe at a time, I'm here to transform your 40s into a vibrant tapestry of wellbeing. Together, let's transform this into a friendship rather than just a book. Are you up for a tasty journey? Yes, I certainly am!

As the author discusses what she has been working for, learn the science, the mysteries, and more. Discover the secrets, the science, and more, As the author shares what she's been fighting for. Low Carb 2024, a revolution in your hands, Where wellness unfolds and a new chapter expands. So turn the page and join this incredible ride, As the Low Carb Queen becomes your

trusted guide. Get ready for a future where vitality thrives, And the author's page becomes the story of your lives.

Introduction

Low Carb 2024 - An Excursion to Wellbeing

I n the high speed universe of wellbeing and nourishment, remaining on the ball is fundamental. Welcome to "Low Carb 2024," a far reaching guide that will drive you into a time of better decisions, dynamic living, and the most recent bits of knowledge on the low-carb way of life.

This isn't simply one more eating regimen; it's a change, a way of life shift intended to strengthen your body, psyche, and soul.

➢ What Looks for You?

As we step into 2024, the universe of low-carb living has advanced and refined itself to meet the one of a kind requirements of people matured 40 and then some.

➢ This book will be your confidant friend on this thrilling excursion:
➢ The Low-Carb Transformation:

Low-carb living has flooded in prominence throughout the long term, and for good explanation. It's not just about shedding those additional pounds; an all encompassing way to deal with health centers around your body's necessities. In this extended excursion, you'll be aware of the most recent patterns, master bits of knowledge, and reasonable tips to make low carb work for you in 2024.

➢ Finding Safe Decisions:

The principal section will direct you through the complexities of a low-carb diet by assisting you with recognizing what's protected to consume

➢ No Sugar, No Issue:

At last, we'll investigate improving without sugar, acquainting you with a universe of sugar substitutes that will entice your taste buds while keeping your carb count low.

➢ Low Carb 2024 is your pass to a better, more vivacious you:

This year is tied in with embracing the fate of low-carb living, remaining at the front of sustenance, and, in particular, carrying on with your best life. We should set out on this excursion together, and make 2024 the year you really flourish.

Chapter 1

Opening ImperativeNess The Low-Carb Diet for Those North of 40+

In our current reality where the journey for a solid, dynamic life never stops, the low-carb diet has arisen as an immortal legend, developing to meet the exceptional necessities of those matured 40 and then some.

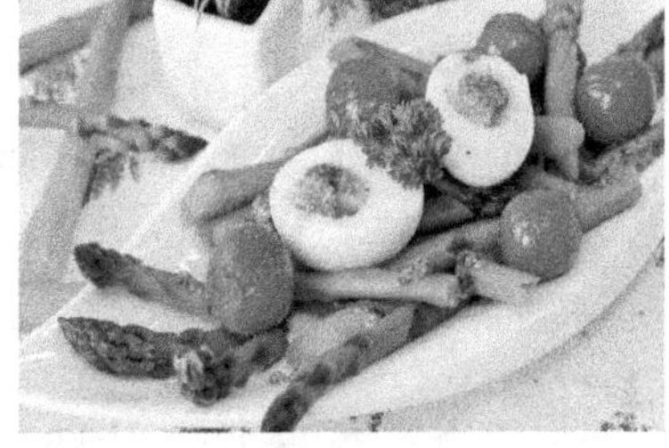

Express farewell to one-size-fits-all eating regimens and welcome a customized approach intended to stimulate your body, brain, and soul.

➤ An Immortal Arrangement:

Low-carb living is definitely not a simple pattern; it's a tried and true arrangement. As you venture as the decades progressed, your wholesome prerequisites advance, and the low-carb diet goes the distance.

It's about higher expectations no matter what, enabling you to settle on decisions that resound with your body's requests.

➤ Welcome to the Low-Carb Way of life:

Low carb isn't simply an eating routine; it's a way of life. It's a significant change in the manner you contemplate food, sustenance, and prosperity.

At 40 and then some, it's not just about shedding pounds; it's tied in with acquiring essentialness, keeping up with smartness, and supporting your resistant framework.

➤ The Wellspring of Youth:

As the years go by, you may be considering the wellspring of youth - a method for looking and feeling your best.

➤ Enter the low-carb diet, your clear-cut advantage:

By lessening carb admission and zeroing in on supplement thick food varieties, you'll encounter expanded energy, work on mental lucidity, and the possibility of a more drawn out, better life.

➤ Weight The executives Made More astute:

Weight the board can be a test as you age. That is where the low-carb diet sparkles. It assists you with shedding undesirable pounds as well as advances muscle conservation, supporting you in keeping an energetic physical make-up.

➤ Glucose and Then some:

For those more than 40, the low-carb diet offers the additional benefit of settling glucose levels, possibly decreasing the gamble of diabetes and improving insulin responsiveness. It's a strong partner as you continue looking for long haul wellbeing.

➢ Heart Wellbeing and Then some:

Low carb isn't just about shedding pounds; it's tied in with focusing on heart wellbeing. By diminishing your carb consumption, you can decrease fatty substances and raise HDL cholesterol, factors that advance a solid cardiovascular framework.

➢ The Low-Carb Excursion Starts:

Your excursion to rejuvenation through the low-carb diet is going to start whether you're looking for feasible weight reduction, upgraded smartness, better glucose control, or essentially a more lively you, the low-carb way of life is your friend on this enabling journey.

Low Carb 2024 is here to direct you, motivate you, and show you the way to a better, more stimulated life.

Prepare to open your imperativeness as we investigate the universe of low-carb living, planned solely for those more than 40.

Raising Life's Stage The Critical Job of Adjusted Sustenance for More established Grown-ups:

As we nimbly age, the meaning of a reasonable eating regimen turns out to be more evident than any other time in recent memory.

For those who've navigated the years and acquired shrewdness, a fair eating routine isn't simply an issue of wellbeing; it's the way to opening the way to imperativeness, life span, and a satisfying life.

➢ An Establishment for Wellbeing:

A fair eating routine isn't simply a dietary routine; it's the bedrock of an energetic presence. It's the encapsulation of the aphorism "the type of food you eat will affect you general health," with each chomp forming the nature of your life. In the brilliant years, a decent eating regimen isn't an extravagance — it's a need.

➢ Supplement Rich Decisions:

As we age, our bodies require an ensemble of supplements to ideally work. A reasonable eating regimen resembles a gold mine of these fundamental components.

It's the specialty of giving your body the nutrients, minerals, and macronutrients that it wants. It's the affirmation that you are filling your body with the secret sauce.

➢ Keeping up with Essentialness:

A fair eating routine is the solution of life, upgrading imperativeness and energy. It's the key to battling age-related weariness and remaining spry.

With the right supplements, you can keep up with the essentialness to pursue your fantasies, investigate new interests, and make lovely recollections.

➢ Saving Mental Clearness:

The mind is the crown gem of your reality. A decent eating routine is its reliable partner, safeguarding mental capability.

Appropriate nourishment can assist with fighting off cognitive decline, reinforce smartness, and sustain the sharpness that permits you to appreciate each experience.

➢ Fortifying the Invulnerable Post:

As we age, our safe framework needs steady help. A reasonable eating regimen gives the ordnance to avert disease and contamination. It's the gatekeeper of your prosperity, bracing your body's protections against the preliminaries of time.

➢ Making preparations for Constant Sicknesses:

The brilliant years accompany their portion of wellbeing challenges. A decent eating routine is your safeguard, safeguarding against

constant illnesses like diabetes, coronary illness, and osteoporosis. It's the way to limit gambling and guarantee a more extended, better life.

➢ Higher expectations without compromise:

In your later years, it's not just about expanding life; it's tied in with improving it. A decent eating routine assists you with flourishing, making consistently an embroidery of prosperity. It's tied in with partaking in your dinners while embracing the insight that life is a valuable gift.

➢ Your Excursion to Satisfaction:

The significance of a reasonable eating regimen for more seasoned grown-ups goes past wellbeing; it's tied in with raising personal satisfaction. It's the foundation whereupon your prosperity is assembled.

With each nibble, you're writing another section, creating a life that is dynamic, dynamic, and rich with encounters.

> As you leave on the excursion of improving with age, recall that a decent eating regimen is your confided in buddy.

The compass guides you toward an existence of imperativeness, lucidity, and satisfaction. It's the key to living your brilliant years without limit, a demonstration of the insight that age is only a number.

Chapter 2

What to Include and Avoid in Your Low Carb Diet

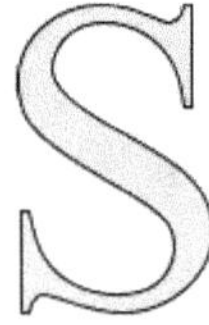

Setting out on a low-carb venture is like venturing into a domain where your decisions become the modelers of your prosperity. Thus, we should discuss what to embrace and what to nimbly evade on your low-carb experience.

➢ Embrace the Greens, Appreciate the Varieties:

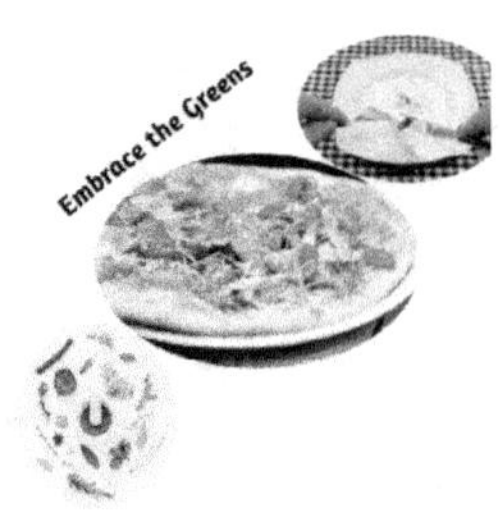

In this low-carb world, your plate is a material, and the greens are the brushstrokes of wellbeing. Jump into mixed greens like spinach, kale, and arugula, embracing their supplement pressed goodness. These veggies add energy to your feasts as well as give fundamental nutrients and minerals.

Presently, we should play with colors! Load up on a range of vegetables like ringer peppers, tomatoes, and broccoli.

Their different tones imply a variety of supplements, making your low-carb plate a work of art of flavors and medical advantages.

➢ Protein Forces to be reckoned with:

Meet your protein forces to be reckoned with - the legends of your low-carb adventure. Lean meats, poultry, fish, and eggs become the dominant focal point, guaranteeing your body gets the fundamental amino acids it aches for.

Plunge into the universe of fish for omega-3 unsaturated fats, advancing heart wellbeing and culinary fulfillment.

➢ Sound Fats:

In this low-carb story, fats are not the foe but rather the partners of flavor and satiety. Avocados, olive oil, and nuts are your confidants in making a sense of taste satisfying ensemble. These solid fats add wealth to your dinners as well as give supported energy, keeping you powered and centered.

➢ Avoid the Sweet Enticements:

Presently, we should explore away from the sweet alarms that can wreck your low-carb mission. Express no to sweet refreshments and select hydrating choices like water, home grown teas, or shining water.

These decisions keep you revived as well as free you from the shackles of pointless sugars.

➢ Careful Carbs:

Carbs, however decreased, are not completely exiled. Embrace the decency of low-carb vegetables and berries. These carb-cognizant decisions add pleasantness to your life as well as convey fundamental supplements without spiking your glucose levels.

➢ Be careful with Refined Grains:

In this low-carb adventure, refined grains are the main adversaries, sneaking in handled food sources and enticing you with void calories.

➢ Express goodbye to white bread, sweet grains, and handled snacks.

All things considered, settle on entire grains like quinoa and cauliflower rice, offering a more supplement thick other option.

➢ Equilibrium and Part Control:

Ok, the specialty of equilibrium and part control - the mainstays of your low-carb realm. Indeed, even with the best fixings, balance is the key. Partake in the wealth of your feasts without indulging, guaranteeing that each chomp is a careful festival of flavors.

➢ Hydration, Your Uncelebrated Yet truly great individual:

In the midst of the low-carb display, hydration remains as your overlooked yet truly great individual. Water extinguishes your thirst as well as helps absorption and supports general prosperity.

Keep a water bottle close by, making hydration a steady friend on your low-carb venture.

➢ Your Low-Carb Experience Is standing by:

As you wind through the decisions of what to incorporate and stay away from in your low-carb diet, recall, this excursion is an individual odyssey. Embrace the greens, relish the proteins, and let sound fats be your partners.

➢ Avoid sweet snares, explore the scene of careful carbs, and be careful with refined grains.

With balance, segment control, and hydration as your compass, your low-carb experience unfurls as a story of energetic well being, delightful dinners, and a restored feeling of prosperity. Partake in each section!

Foods to avoid and the reasons behind their exclusion in a low-carb diet for older adults

In the exhilarating undertaking of taking on a low-carb way of life for more seasoned grown-ups, it's crucial to embrace the right food varieties as well as to say goodbye to the dietary miscreants that can impede your excursion to wellbeing and essentialness.

How about we investigate the food varieties to stay away from and the convincing purposes for their avoidance in your low-carb diet.

1. Refined Sugars: The Sweet Harm.

Sugar is the enchanting saboteur that entices your taste buds while unleashing destruction on your wellbeing.

By dispensing with refined sugars from your eating regimen, you'll keep up with stable glucose levels, advance weight reduction, and lessen the gamble of diabetes.

2. White Bread and Pasta: Carb Guilty parties.

White bread and pasta are handled, refined starch bombs that send your glucose on a rollercoaster ride.

These carb guilty parties offer minimal concerning sustenance and can prompt energy crashes and weight gain.

3. Sweet Tidbits and Soft drinks: Void Calories.

Sweet tidbits and soft drinks are a definitive void of calorie extravagances. They spike your glucose as well as offer minimal nourishing benefits. By barring these sweet enjoyments, you'll take a monster jump toward a better, more adjusted diet.

4. Potatoes: Dull Risks

Potatoes, however darling, are dull dangers that can rapidly crash your low-carb endeavors.

They're high in starches and can prompt undesirable weight gain and glucose changes.

5. Cereals and Breakfast Bars: Stowed away Sugars

Many breakfast cereals and bars are misleadingly weighed down with stowed sugars. Perusing names is fundamental, as these apparently blameless items can send your glucose taking off.

6. Handled Food sources: Substance Mess

Handled food varieties are famous for containing stowed away sugars, undesirable fats, and a variety of counterfeit added substances.
Staying away from these compound entanglements is critical for protecting your wellbeing and essentialness.

7. Organic products High in Sugar: Proceed Cautiously

While natural products offer fundamental supplements, some are higher in sugar than others.

Limit your admission of natural products like bananas, grapes, and dried natural products to stay away from superfluous carb consumption.

8. Natural product Juices: Fluid Sugar.

Natural product juices, regardless of their wellbeing radiance, are much of the time minimal more than fluid sugar.

They miss the mark on fiber and supplements tracked down in entire leafy foods lead to glucose spikes.

9. Lager: Fluid Carbs

Lager is a fluid wellspring of carbs, and not the great kind.

It's calorie-thick and can subvert your low-carb progress.

10. Inexpensive Food: The Snare of Comfort

Cheap food might be advantageous, yet it's normally rich in undesirable carbs and low in dietary benefit.

Keeping away from these dietary snares is fundamental for keeping a low-carb way of life.

➢ The Low-Carb Commitment:

By saying goodbye to these dietary enemies, you're not trying to say no to purge calories and undesirable carbs.

You're expressing yes to a future loaded up with wellbeing, imperativeness, and the opportunity to partake in a daily existence liberated from glucose spikes and energy crashes.

The rejection of these food sources in your low-carb diet for more seasoned grown-ups is a purposeful decision to impact your life into an account of wellbeing and liveliness.

It's the commitment of a better tomorrow, one that you compose with each careful dinner decision you make.

Chapter 3

Overseeing Calories and Nourishing Data - Your Recipe for Wellbeing

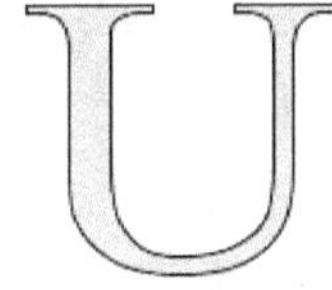

nderstanding Calorie The directors and Part Control- Your Way to Engaged Eating Drink to the core of your low- carb adventure, where we dive into the craft of calorie board and the fragile equilibrium of price control.

This part is commodity other than figures; it's tied in with recovering your control over your plate and sustaining your body with delicacy.

Calorie The directors Filling Your Essentialness Calories are the energy that keeps your body's motor handling.

In this section, you will reveal the mystifications of calorie operation, guaranteeing that you consume the perfect proportion of energy for your day to day needs.

There is really no need to concentrate on counting each calorie; it's tied in with understanding the job calories play in your essentialness.

delicate exercise The Craft of Part Control. Member control is your distinct advantage in the charge for a decent eating authority.

> ➢ It's tied in with figuring out the perfect balance among fulfillment and control:

In this section, you will come amazing at member control, so you can partake in your feasts without feeling denied.

Advanced prospects when in distrustfulness The Way to Fulfillment With member control, there is actually no need to concentrate on eating less; it's tied in with eating expertise.

This part directs you to concentrate on better norms when in distrustfulness, guaranteeing that each chomp is loaded with supplements, flavors, and fulfillment. It's the pathway to righteous shamefaced pleasure Careful Eating Appreciating Each Chomp.

Careful eating is an exposure in this section. It's tied in with delighting each mouthful, connecting every one of your faculties, and really valuing your food.

By being available at each feast, you can upgrade your eating experience, perceive completion signals, and typically exercise member control.

The Brilliant Rule Equilibrium and multifariousness negativing your feasts with different supplements is the brilliant rule:

This section delineates how colorful food sources complete one another, giving the right equilibrium of carbs, proteins, and fats to keep you satisfied and empowered.

Another Relationship with Food Sustenance Over Extravagance This section will make a significant change in your relationship with food.

There is really no need to concentrate on roistering or confining; It's tied in with supporting your body and embracing a careful way to deal with eating.

By understanding part control and calorie operation, you gain the occasion to go with conscious opinions, appreciate your feasts, and assume responsibility for your good:

The Force of Decision Your Low- Carb Excursion Understanding calorie the board and part control is not simply a section in your excursion; it's the foundation of your engaged eating.

With this information, you will explore your low- carb way of life with certainty, realizing that each gash you take is a conscious decision, powering your way to good, essentialness, and a diurnal actuality brimming with scrumptious hassles.

Your Way to Engaged Eating Starts Then Section 3 is further than data; it's your way to enable eating:

The assistant opens the secrets of calories and parts, guaranteeing that your low-carb adventure is not just about what you eat, yet the way in which you eat it.

With this information close by, you have the capability to shape your ideal low-carb way of life, each careful and fulfilling chomp in turn. Drink to the macrocosm of deliberate and engaged eating.

Understanding Calorie The executives and Part Control - Your Way to Engaged Eating

Welcome to the core of your low-carb venture, where we dive into the craft of calorie board and the fragile equilibrium of price control.

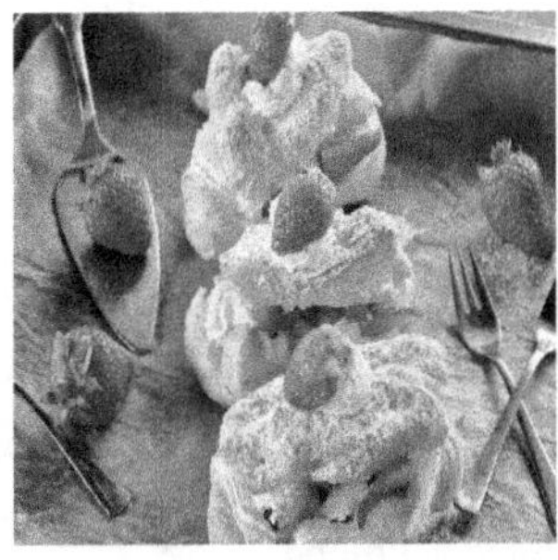

This part is something other than numbers; it's tied in with recovering your control over your plate and sustaining your body with accuracy.

Calorie The Executives Filling Your Essentialness:

Calories are the fuel that keeps your body's motor running:

In this section, you'll reveal the mysteries of calorie management, guaranteeing that you consume the perfect proportion of energy for your day to day needs.

There's really no need to focus on counting each calorie; it's tied in with understanding the job calories play in your essentialness.

➤ Difficult exercise: The Craft of Part Control:

Segment control is your distinct advantage in the mission for a decent eating regimen. It's tied in with figuring out the perfect balance among fulfillment and control.

In this section, you'll become amazing at segment control, so you can partake in your dinners without feeling denied.

➤ Higher expectations when in doubt the way to fulfillment:

With segment control, there's actually no need to focus on eating less; it's tied in with eating savvy.
This part directs you to focus on better standards when in doubt, guaranteeing that each chomp is loaded with supplements, flavors, and fulfillment.

➤ It's the pathway to righteous guilty pleasure:
➤ Careful Eating: Appreciating Each Chomp.

Careful eating is a disclosure in this section. It's tied in with relishing each nibble, connecting every one of your faculties, and really valuing your food.

By being available at each feast, you can upgrade your eating experience, perceive completion signals, and normally practice segment control.

Disclosing the Insider facts of Nourishing Data

Step into, where the drape ascends on the confounding universe of dietary data. This isn't simply information; it's the code to a better, more educated way regarding eating.

Plan to open the secrets of macronutrients, micronutrients, and the power they hold over your prosperity.

➢ The Higher perspective: Dietary Data Outline:
➢ In this part, we'll lay out the 10,000 foot view of wholesome data:

You'll grasp the central members in your eating routine, from macronutrients like carbs, proteins, and fats to the micronutrients - nutrients and minerals.
This isn't just about counting; it's tied in with appreciating the structure blocks of your wellbeing.

➢ Protein: Your Body's Partner.

Protein becomes the overwhelming focus. It's not only a supplement; it's your body's partner in building, fixing, and keeping up with.

In this section, you'll dive into the significance of protein, how it upholds muscle strength, and holds your hunger within proper limits, making it your go-to supplement for manageable prosperity.

➢ Fiber The Stomach related Dynamo:

Fiber isn't simply roughage; the stomach related dynamo holds your stomach wellbeing in line.

In this section, you'll uncover the pivotal job of fiber in weight, the executives, absorption, and even glucose control.
It's not just about consistency; it's tied in with embracing this superpower for an energetic life.

> ➤ Sugars: Figuring out the Great and the Awful:
> ➤ Carbs are a hotly debated issue:

This section will direct you to separate between the great and the awful carbs, so you can go with informed decisions.

There's no need to focus on hardship; it's tied in with choosing carbs that line up with your wellbeing objectives.

> ➤ Fats The Solid Fat Disclosure:

The discussion on fats is developing. In this part, you'll discover that not all fats are your adversaries.

Solid fats are your body's partners in advancing generally wellbeing, from supporting your body to making your feasts seriously fulfilling. It's not necessary to focus on staying away from fats; it's tied in with embracing the right kind.

> ➤ Sugars The Secret Saboteurs:

Sugar can be a shrewd enemy. This section uncovers the secret sugars prowling in regular food sources and beverages.

By understanding sugar and its other options, you gain the ability to go with informed decisions and safeguard your wellbeing.

➤ Balance: The Wholesome Orchestra:

This part isn't about numbers; it's about balance. The orchestra of supplements structure the soundtrack of your life. It's tied in with understanding how macronutrients and micronutrients work as one, guaranteeing your body flourishes.

➤ The Recipe of Health Starts:

your recipe for health. It's not simply data; it's the way to grasp your eating regimen's most crucial components. With this information, you're prepared to settle on informed choices, making a life that is better, more enthusiastic, and seriously fulfilling.

Welcome to the universe of wholesome data, where your decisions aren't just about what you eat, yet about how you fuel your wellbeing and essentialness, each supplement in turn.

Chapter 4

Opening the Force of Fundamental Nutrients and Minerals for 2024

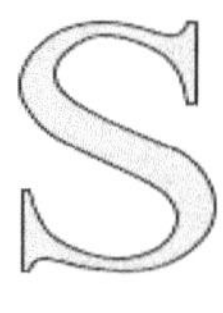 tep into the universe, where the entryway opens to uncover the basic job of fundamental nutrients and minerals in your low-carb venture.

This section isn't just about supplements; it's tied in with opening the keys to a better, more energetic life in the year 2024.

➤ Vitamin A The Visionary:

Vitamin A takes the spotlight, exhibiting its visionary powers. In this section, you'll reveal how vitamin A backings your eyes, skin, and resistant framework.

It's not just about carrots; it's about the reasonable vision and brilliant wellbeing it brings to your life.

➤ Bone Wellbeing: Nutrients D and K as the Unique Team:

Bone wellbeing is imperative, and nutrients D and K are the unique team that guarantees your bones areas of strength for stay.

In this section, you'll disentangle how these nutrients work in collaboration to help your skeletal framework and then some. It's not just about milk; it's about the groundwork of your prosperity.

➢ Nutrients C and E The Cell reinforcement Vindicators:

The cancer prevention agent vindicators, nutrients C and E, act the hero. In this section, you'll investigate how these nutrients safeguard your cells, battle maturing, and sustain your resistant framework. It's not just about oranges; it's about the safeguards of your body against the progression of time.

➢ B-Nutrients: The Energy Devotees:

B-Nutrients are the energy devotees inside you. In this part, you'll get a handle on their job in changing food into fuel, supporting mind capability, and helping your general essentialness. It's not just about grains; it's tied in with being vivacious at each phase of life.

➢ Mineral Wonders Iron, Calcium, and then some:

Minerals are the overlooked yet truly great individuals of your eating routine, from iron, fundamental for oxygen transport, to calcium, pivotal for bone wellbeing. In this part, you'll see the value in the meaning of minerals and how they enhance your life. It's not just about supplements; minerals are central for a vigorous body.

➤ Folate The Recovery Maestro:

Folate makes that big appearance as the recovery maestro. In this section, you'll find its part in DNA arrangement, tissue development, and generally speaking wellbeing. It's not just about green vegetables; it's about the insider facts of recovery.

➤ Balance The Agreeable Mix:

This section is an ensemble of fundamental nutrients and minerals, each having its extraordinary influence to form a solid life. It's   just about supplements; it's about balance, guaranteeing your body gets the agreeable mix of nutrients and minerals it aches for.

➤ Your Excursion to Wellbeing Starts:

your doorway to wellbeing. It's not simply data; it's the manual for grasping the meaning of nutrients and minerals in your wellbeing process. With this information, you're prepared to settle on purposeful decisions, creating a life that is better, more vivacious, and really fulfilling.

Welcome to the universe of fundamental nutrients and minerals for 2024, where your decisions aren't just about what you eat, yet about how you clear the way to an existence of imperativeness and prosperity.

A fresh look at critical vitamins and minerals for those aged 40+ in 2024

In Part 4, we leave on an excursion into the universe of basic nutrients and minerals, offering a new viewpoint for those matured 40+ in the year 2024. This part is something beyond supplements; it's a passage to essentialness, prosperity, and the insight of informed decisions.

➤ Vitamin A: The Ever-enduring Visionary:

Vitamin A becomes the overwhelming focus, and its job as an ever-enduring visionary is revealed. In this part, you'll find how vitamin A backings your eyes, skin, and safe framework as you improve with age.

It's not just about carrots; it's about clear vision and brilliant wellbeing, enduring great into your 40s and then some.

➤ Bone Wellbeing: The Power Couple of Nutrients D and K:

Bone wellbeing is a long lasting excursion, and nutrients D and K structure the tough power team that guarantees your bones major areas of strength for stay.

In this part, you'll uncover their synergistic job in supporting your skeletal framework and then some.

It's not just about milk; it's tied in with keeping up with the underpinning of your prosperity as you enter your 40s and then some.

> Nutrients C and E: Improving with age with Cancer prevention agent Partners: Improving with age is a workmanship, and nutrients C and E are your partners all the while.

In this part, you'll investigate how these nutrients safeguard your phones, battle maturing, and brace your resistant framework, offering you the key to remaining lively as you become older.

It's not just about oranges; it's tied in with embracing the safeguards of your body against the progression of time.

> B-Nutrients The Wellspring of Energy:

Energy is a fortune at whatever stage in life, and B-Nutrients are your wellspring of essentialness.

In this section, you'll comprehend their vital job in changing food into fuel, supporting cerebrum capability, and improving your general energy levels as you embrace your 40s and then some. It's not just about grains; it's tied in with remaining enthusiastic and brimming with life.

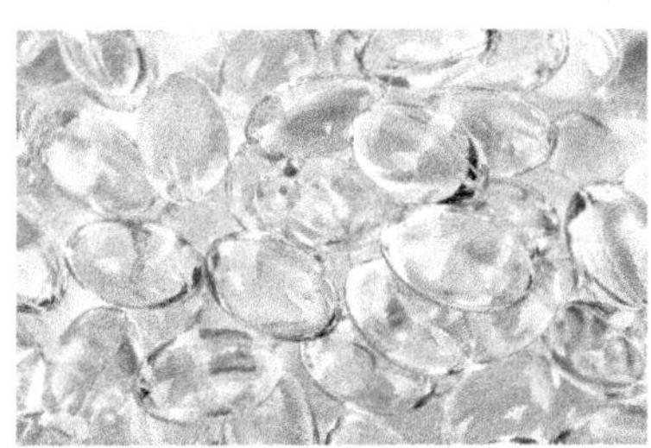

➤ Mineral Wonders Iron, Calcium, and Then some:

Minerals are the overlooked yet truly great individuals of your eating regimen, and as you arrive at your 40s and then some, their significance just develops.

From iron, fundamental for oxygen transport, to calcium, crucial for bone wellbeing, this part uncovers how minerals advance your life and keep up with your imperativeness. It's not just about supplements; embracing the minerals are fundamental for a vigorous body as you improve with age.

➤ Folate: The Recovery Trained professional:

Folate accepts the spotlight as the recovery trained professional, directing your body's recharging.

In this section, you'll find out about its part in DNA development, tissue development, and by and large wellbeing, furnishing you with the way to feeling energetic and restored very much into your 40s and then some. It's not just about green vegetables; it's about the mysteries of recovery.

➢ Balance: The Way to Imperishable Health:

This section is an orchestra of fundamental nutrients and minerals, each having its remarkable impact in making a day to day existence out of ever-enduring wellbeing.

It's not just about supplements; it's about balance, guaranteeing your body gets the amicable mix of nutrients and minerals to keep you imperative and flourishing in your 40s and then some.

➢ Your Ever-enduring Health Excursion Starts:

isn't simply data; it's your entryway to ever-enduring wellbeing. It's the manual for understanding the meaning of basic nutrients and minerals as you enter your 40s and then some.

With this information, you're prepared to settle on informed decisions, making a life that is loaded up with imperativeness, prosperity, and the insight of imperishable wellbeing.

Welcome to the universe of basic nutrients and minerals for those matured 40+ in 2024, where your decisions aren't just about what you eat, yet about how you keep on embracing an existence of essentialness and prosperity.

Guaranteeing Your Healthful Prerequisites are Met Through Diet

We unwind the craft of ensuring that your nourishing necessities are met through your everyday eating regimen.

This section is something other than eating; it's your guide to a day to day existence overflowing with wellbeing, imperativeness, and the certainty that your decisions line up with your requirements.

➤ Difficult exercise: The Center of Wholesome Adequacy:

Adjusting your eating regimen is the way to guaranteeing your wholesome prerequisites are met. In this part, you'll gain proficiency with the specialty of making dinners that give every one of the fundamental supplements your body aches for. It's not just about food; it's tied in with organizing an ensemble of wellbeing.

➤ Expand: The Sorcery of Assortment:

Monotony wears on the soul in your eating regimen, the enchanted wand ensures nourishing adequacy.

This part will show you how embracing various food sources guarantees that you get a wide range of nutrients, minerals, and supplements.

It's not just about tedium; it's about the experience of flavors, surfaces, and sustenance.

➤ Careful Eating: Appreciating the Experience:

Careful eating is the highlight of this section. It's tied in with appreciating each chomp, being available at your feasts, and grasping your body's signals.

By rehearsing careful eating, you can tweak your decisions to guarantee that your wholesome necessities are met. It's not just about utilization; it's about a cognizant association with your body's necessities.

➢ Mark Proficiency Interpreting Food Names:

Food marks can be your partners in the mission for healthful adequacy. In this part, you'll turn into a name investigator, figuring out how to translate the data on bundling to pursue informed decisions. It's not just about items; it's about the ability to understand what you're consuming.

➢ Segment Dominance: The Goldilocks Guideline:

Segment control is something other than abstaining from indulging; about guaranteeing you're eating the perfect add up to meet your

wholesome prerequisites. This part dives into the Goldilocks standard, finding the piece that is perfect for your body. It's not just about less or more; it's about the ideal equilibrium.

➢ Supplementation: The Additional Mile:

Enhancements can be your partners in gathering nourishing prerequisites, particularly assuming your eating regimen misses the mark in specific regions.

This section gives knowledge into when and how to utilize enhancements to overcome any barrier. It's not just about pills; it's tied in with guaranteeing your healthful necessities are met.

➤ The Outline for Wholesome Adequacy:

This section isn't just about keeping a bunch of guidelines; about creating an outline for dietary adequacy lines up with your life and your extraordinary necessities.

With this information, you'll have the ability to pursue intentional decisions, guaranteeing that your wholesome necessities are met through diet. It's not just about food; It's about the satisfaction of your body's requirements.

➤ Your Excursion to Wholesome Adequacy Starts:

Isn't simply data; it's your excursion to wholesome adequacy.
It's the manual for figuring out the fragile specialty of adjusting your eating routine, expanding your decisions, rehearsing careful eating, translating marks, dominating parts, and utilizing supplements when essential.

➤ With this information, you're ready to guarantee that your dietary prerequisites are met, creating a day to day existence loaded up with wellbeing, essentialness, and the certainty that you're sustaining your body perfectly:

Welcome to the universe of healthful adequacy, where your decisions aren't just about what you eat, yet about how you guarantee your prosperity through your everyday eating routine.

Chapter 5

Guaranteeing Your Nourishing Prerequisites are Met Through Diet

In Part 5, we disentangle the specialty of ensuring that your wholesome necessities are met through your everyday eating routine. BThis section is something other than eating; it's your guide to a day to day existence overflowing with wellbeing, essentialness, and the certainty that your decisions line up with your requirements.

➤ Difficult exercise: The Center of Healthful Adequacy:

Adjusting your eating routine is the way to guarantee your dietary necessities are met. In this part, you'll get familiar with the craft of making dinners that give every one of the fundamental supplements your body needs. It's not just about food; it's tied in with coordinating an ensemble of wellbeing.

➤ Enhance: The Sorcery of Assortment:

Monotony wears on the soul in your eating routine, the enchanted wand ensures nourishing adequacy.

This part will show you how embracing various food sources guarantees that you get a wide range of nutrients, minerals, and supplements.

It's not just about tedium; it's about the experience of flavors, surfaces, and sustenance.

➤ Careful Eating: Relishing the Experience:

Careful eating is the focal point of this section. It's tied in with relishing each chomp, being available at your feasts, and grasping your body's signals. By rehearsing careful eating, you can calibrate your decisions to guarantee that your nourishing necessities are met.

It's not just about utilization; it's about a cognizant association with your body's requirements.

➤ Name Proficiency: Interpreting Food Marks:

Food names can be your partners in the mission for healthful adequacy. In this part, you'll turn into a mark analyst, figuring out how to translate the data on bundling to go with informed decisions. It's not just about items; it's about the ability to understand what you're consuming.

➤ Segment Dominance: The Goldilocks Standard:

Segment control is something other than abstaining from indulging; about guaranteeing you're eating the perfect add up to meet your dietary necessities.

This part dives into the Goldilocks standard, finding the piece that is perfect for your body. It's not just about less or more; it's about the ideal equilibrium.

➤ Supplementation The Additional Mile:

Enhancements can be your partners in gathering healthful necessities, particularly assuming your eating routine misses the mark in specific regions.

This section gives understanding into when and how to utilize enhancements to overcome any barrier. It's not just about pills; it's tied in with guaranteeing your healthful necessities are met.

➤ The Diagram for Nourishing Adequacy:

This section isn't just about keeping a bunch of guidelines; about creating an outline for dietary adequacy lines up with your life and your novel requirements. With this information, you'll have the ability to settle on purposeful decisions, guaranteeing that your healthful prerequisites are met

through diet. It's not just about food; it's about the satisfaction of your body's requirements.

➤ Your Excursion to Healthful Adequacy Starts:

It's your excursion to dietary adequacy. It's the manual for grasping the fragile craft of adjusting your eating regimen, expanding your decisions, rehearsing careful eating, disentangling marks, dominating parts, and utilizing supplements when essential.

With this information, you're ready to guarantee that your wholesome prerequisites are met, making a daily existence loaded up with wellbeing, essentialness, and the certainty that you're supporting your body perfectly:

Welcome to the universe of wholesome adequacy, where your decisions aren't just about what you eat, yet about how you guarantee your prosperity through your day to day diet.

The Essential Job of L-ascorbic acid in Supporting In general Wellbeing

We plunge profoundly into the imperative job of L-ascorbic acid, a supplement that fills in as the key part for generally wellbeing. This section is something other than data; it's a disclosure of how this modest nutrient is a foundation for your prosperity and imperativeness.

➢ Insusceptible Fortifier Your Most memorable Line of Safeguard:

L-ascorbic acid isn't simply a nutrient; it's your most memorable line of guard against illnesses. In this section, you'll find how it reinforces your resistant framework, assisting your body with combatting contaminations and remaining tough against current difficulties. It's not just about squeezed orange; it's tied in with building an impervious fort against ailments.

➢ Collagen Maker The Way to Energetic Skin Areas of strength:

Collagen is the key to young skin and vigorous joints. L-ascorbic acid plays the job of a collagen maker, ensuring your skin stays flexible and your joints stay coordinated. In this

part, you'll investigate how it's not just about creams and serums; it's tied in with embracing the regular wellspring of youth inside

➢ Cancer prevention agent Champion: Shielding Cells from Oxidative Pressure:

In a world loaded up with free revolutionaries, L-ascorbic acid turns into your cell reinforcement champion. It safeguards your cells and DNA against oxidative pressure, protecting your general wellbeing.

In this section, you'll figure out how it's not just about supplements; it's tied in with saddling the regular safeguard your body offers.

➢ Heart Wellbeing Partner: Supporting Your Cardiovascular Framework:

L-ascorbic acid isn't just about citrus natural products; it's additionally about heart wellbeing. This section dives into its job in keeping up with sound veins and advancing generally speaking cardiovascular prosperity. It's not just about dietary decisions; about a supplement adds to a strong cardiovascular framework.

➤ Mental Essentialness Your Mental Help:

Mental deftness is a valued resource in the present speedy world. L-ascorbic acid turns into your partner in keeping up with mental essentialness. In this part, you'll find how it upholds mental capability, keeping you sharp, engaged, and prepared to handle life's difficulties. It's not just about the mind working out; a supplement feeds your smartness.

➤ The Ensemble of Wellbeing L-ascorbic acid's Diverse Job:

L-ascorbic acid isn't simply a nutrient; an ensemble of wellbeing coordinates health from different points. It fortifies your resistant framework, sustains young skin and joints, shields against free revolutionaries, upholds heart wellbeing, and lifts mental imperativeness. It's not just around one-layered wellbeing; embracing a supplement assumes a diverse part in your prosperity.

➤ Your Excursion to Ideal Wellbeing Starts:

It's your excursion to opening the capability of L-ascorbic acid for your general wellbeing. With this information, you're prepared to settle on informed decisions, guaranteeing that you embrace this supplement as an urgent component in your quest for wellbeing, imperativeness, and flexibility in the cutting edge world.

Welcome to the existence where your decisions aren't just about what you eat, yet about how you enable your general wellbeing through the exceptional impact of L-ascorbic acid.

The Best Wellsprings of L-ascorbic acid for Your Body in 2024 - Sustenance for the Advanced Age

In this section, we leave on an excursion to investigate the best wellsprings of L-ascorbic acid, reclassifying the manner in which you support your body in 2024.

This is something beyond dietary exhortation; it's your manual for mixing your advanced existence with the fundamental L-ascorbic acid your body wants.

➢ Citrus Sensations Oranges, Lemons, and Limes:

Citrus organic products have forever been exemplary wellsprings of L-ascorbic acid. In this section, you'll rediscover the ageless allure of oranges, lemons, and limes. They're not simply natural products; they're your fiery associates making a course for wellbeing.

➢ Past Citrus Berries, Kiwi, and Papaya:

Now is the ideal time to go past the works of art. Berries, kiwi, and papaya become the dominant focal point as rich wellsprings of L-ascorbic acid. In this part, you'll discover that L-ascorbic acid isn't just about oranges; it's tied in with embracing a rainbow of flavors, varieties, and supplements.

➢ Garden Goodness: Chime Peppers and Broccoli:

Your nursery is a mother lode of L-ascorbic acid. Ringer peppers and broccoli arise as nursery goodness that can supercharge your wellbeing. In this section, you'll find that your L-ascorbic acid sources aren't simply organic products; they're vegetables that bring tone, crunch, and sustenance to your plate.

➢ The Force of Spices Parsley and Thyme.

Spices are culinary legends that likewise sneak up all of a sudden. Parsley and thyme take the spotlight in this part, uncovering how they can raise your dishes and your wellbeing. It's not just about flavors; embracing spices sustains your body in each nibble.

➢ Present day Superfood Acerola Cherry.

In the cutting edge age, superfoods have done something significant, and the Acerola cherry is a rising star. This section acquaints you with the superfood status of Acerola cherries, displaying how they're something beyond natural products; they're the advanced ammo for your wellbeing.

➢ Supplements Overcoming any issues:

Supplements become the extension to guarantee you meet your day to day L-ascorbic acid necessities. In this section, you'll comprehend when and how to integrate supplements into your eating routine to fill the holes. It's not just about pills; it's tied in with guaranteeing that your body gets the L-ascorbic acid it needs.

➢ Your Excursion to Ideal Wellbeing Through L-ascorbic acid Starts:

Isn't simply data; it's your excursion to finding the best wellsprings of L-ascorbic acid for your body in 2024. With this information, you're prepared to settle on informed decisions, guaranteeing that you embrace

Chapter 6

Uncovering the Carnivore Diet in 2024 - A New Viewpoint on Sustenance

Where we strip back the layers of the Carnivore Diet in 2024, offering a new viewpoint on nourishment. This is something beyond an eating regimen; a disclosure of a way of life's causing disturbances in the realm of wellbeing and health.

➤ Straightforward About Creature Food sources:

The Meat eater Diet returns you to rudiments, zeroing in on creature food varieties as the essential wellspring of sustenance. In this section, you'll investigate how it's not just about patterns; embracing an eating regimen flourishes with the base embodiment of life.

➤ The No-Plant Oddity All Meat, No Greens:

In our current reality where plant-based slims down are much of the time commended, the Meat eater Diet turns the tables, underlining no plants by any means. This section dives into the no-plant oddity, making sense of how it's not just about servings of mixed greens; it's about the force of unadulterated creature sustenance.

➤ Meat-Just Outlook The Advntages and Contentions:

The meat-just outlook is at the core of the Carnivore Diet, offering extraordinary advantages and blending discussions. In this section, you'll comprehend how it's not just about meat; it's about the possibility to change your wellbeing and challenge assumptions.

➤ Effortlessness and Virtue: The Appeal of Meat eater:

Effortlessness and virtue are the signs of the Carnivore Diet, pursuing an appealing decision for those looking for a clear way to deal with sustenance. In this section, you'll investigate how it's not just about difficulties; it's about the charm of an eating regimen that is pretty much as basic and unadulterated as it gets.

➤ Exploring Wholesome Worries: What the Carnivore Diet Offers:

Wholesome worries are frequently at the front while considering an eating regimen that bars whole nutrition types. This section reveals insight into what the Meat eater Diet offers concerning sustenance, exhibiting that it's not just about restrictions; it's tied in with settling on determined decisions.

> ➢ Your Excursion to Meat eater Starts:

It's your excursion to reveal the Carnivore Diet in 2024. With this information, you're prepared to pursue informed decisions, investigating a way of life that is having a momentous effect on the universe of wellbeing and nourishment. Welcome to the existence where your decisions aren't just about what you eat; It's tied in with embracing another point of view on nourishment, introducing the Carnivore Diet as a likely pathway to wellbeing and health.

An updated introduction to the carnivore diet and its potential benefits in 2024

A Refreshed Prologue to the Meat eater Diet and Its Possible Advantages in 2024 - A Brief look into the Development of Sustenance Welcome to a cutting edge investigation of the Carnivore Diet, where we rethink the discussion in 2024:

This section is something beyond a presentation; it's an excursion into the development of sustenance, offering new viewpoints on the well established practice of devouring creature food sources.

➢ The Flesh eater Diet More or less: A Change in outlook:

In a world immersed with dietary decisions, the Meat eater Diet remains as a change in outlook. It's a straightforward methodology where creature food varieties take the middle stage. In this part, you'll plunge into its pith, perceiving that it's not only an eating routine; it's a striking rethinking of nourishment.

➢ The No-Plant Catch 22: Sustenance Without Greens:

The Carnivore Diet challenges the standard way of thinking of embracing salad greens and plant-based slims down. Here, the oddity lies in its absolute rejection of plants. In this section, you'll disentangle the no-plant mystery, recognizing that it's not just about servings of mixed greens; it's tied in with investigating the force of creature based sustenance.

➢ The All-Meat Outlook: Advantages and Debates in the Cutting edge Time:

An all-meat mentality could appear to be an extreme takeoff from adjusted slims down, yet it conveys one of a kind advantages and ignites debate. In 2024, this section will direct you through the developing story encompassing the Flesh Eater Diet, uncovering that it's not just about meats; about embracing a way of life that rocks the boat.

➢ Back to Straightforwardness and Virtue: The Charm of Flesh eater in a Perplexing World:

In our speedy, confounded world, the appeal of straightforwardness and immaculateness can't be undervalued. The Carnivore Diet offers unequivocally that. It's tied in with getting back to the essential demonstration of devouring what the earth gives - creature food sources.

In this section, you'll get a handle on the fact that it's not just about complexities; about the attraction of an eating routine that offers straightforwardness and virtue.

➢ Adjusting Nourishing Worries: What the Flesh eater Diet Offers Today:

Nourishing worries normally emerge when a whole nutrition type, like plants, is barred. The Flesh eater Diet has seen an advancement in its methodology, tending to these worries. In 2024, you'll acquire experiences into what the Carnivore Diet offers regarding nourishment, figuring out that it's not just about impediments; it's about determined decisions.

➢ Your Advanced Excursion into the Meat eater Diet Starts:

It's the commencement of your advanced excursion into the Meat eater Diet in 2024. With this information, you're prepared to pursue informed decisions, investigating a way of life that is adjusting and flourishing in the developing scene of nourishment.

Welcome to the existence where your decisions aren't just about what you eat; it's tied in with embracing a refreshed prologue to the Carnivore Diet, opening ways to the potential advantages it offers in the unique domain of wellbeing and health.

Integrating Creature Based Food sources into a Low-Carb Diet for Everybody

In the realm of dietary decisions, the low-carb diet has acquired conspicuousness for its capability to advance weight reduction, settle glucose levels, and back generally speaking wellbeing. Yet, shouldn't something be said about the individuals who treasure their affection for creatures and put together food sources while with respect to this excursion?

Uplifting news: a low-carb diet can be custom fitted to suit the desires of carnivores and creature food devotees the same.

➢ The Low-Carb, Creature Based Mix A Nourishing Force to be reckoned with:

We should reexamine the idea of a low-carb diet, featuring the consistent joining of creature based food varieties. In this methodology, you'll find that it's not just about prohibitive carbs; it's tied in with embracing the nourishing force to be reckoned with of creature food varieties.

➢ Protein Palooza: Creature Food sources for Satiety and Muscle Wellbeing:

Protein becomes the dominant focal point in this version of the low-carb diet. Creature based sources like lean meats, poultry, and fish become the groundwork of your dinners. In this methodology, you'll figure out that it's not just about plates of mixed greens and vegetables; it's about satiety, muscle wellbeing, and relishing the delectability of creature protein.

➢ Fat for Flavor and Satiety: Embracing Creature Fats:

Creature fats, frequently ignored, offer an enticing aspect to the low-carb diet. From margarine to fat, these fats add both flavor and a feeling of completion to your feasts. In this methodology, you'll understand that it's not just about vegetable oils; it's tied in with enjoying the extravagance of creature based fats.

> ➤ Investigating Assortment: From Hamburger to Buffalo, Chicken to Fish.

The excellence of creature based food varieties is their variety. From the wealth of hamburger to the lean effortlessness of chicken, the seas' abundance of fish to the heartiness of buffalo, there's a universe of choices to investigate. In this methodology, you'll uncover that it's not just about tedious dinners; about a sense of taste constantly energized and fulfilled.

> ➤ Exploring Wholesome Worries: Tracking down the Equilibrium.

A low-carb, creature based diet expects consideration regarding wholesome equilibrium. This approach digs into overseeing large scale and micronutrients, guaranteeing you address your body's issues.

> ➤ In this methodology, you'll perceive that it's not just about carbs; about a smart equilibrium ensures your prosperity:

An Eating regimen for the Carnivore on a fundamental level: Your Customized Excursion This isn't just about squeezing into a shape; about creating an eating routine that reverberates with the meat eater in you. Whether you're an enthusiastic admirer of steak, fish, or poultry, the low-carb, creature based diet permits you to tweak your feasts.

In this methodology, you'll embrace that it's not just about unbending rules; it's about a customized venture into the universe of creature food sources.

> An Excursion of Flavor and Imperativeness Starts:

Integrating creature based food varieties into a low-carb diet for everybody isn't simply a dietary decision; it's an investigation of flavors, a festival of satiety, and an excursion into imperativeness. With this methodology, you're prepared to pursue informed decisions, enhancing your low-carb diet with the exquisite decency of creature based food varieties. Welcome to the existence where your dietary decisions aren't just about limitation; they're tied in with enjoying the superb mix of low-carb, creature based fulfillment.

Chapter 7

Solid Banquet Contemplations for Every Occasion

Relish the Assortment of Incredible Eating In the domain of culinary examination, the possible results are enormous, and your trip into solid banquet contemplations for every occasion will begin.

This isn't just about routine eating; about a weaving of tastes and experiences take exceptional consideration of every single preview of your life.

➤ Morning Brightness Breakfast Display:

As the sun graces the horizon, breakfast lays out the energy for your day.

It's not just about grain; it's about a morning dinner display with dynamic smoothie bowls, avocado toast, and fluffy omelets that invite you with a gathering of flavors and enhancements.

➤ Early afternoon Encounters Early evening Delights:

Right when early evening appears, your feeling of taste wants insight. It's not just about sandwiches; it's about early afternoon delights like supporting plates of leafy greens, liberal soups, and tasty wraps that transport your taste buds to new horizons, making lunch a thrilling endeavor for your resources.

➤ Evening Quietness Goody Time Brilliance:

Amidst the early afternoon calm, snack time is your shelter. It's not just about chips; it's about snack time quality with new veggie platters, smooth yogurt parfaits, and energy-assisting nuts that embed your day with centrality, changing average minutes into more modest than typical celebrations.

➤ Dinnertime Elegance: Night Celebrations.

Evenings are for class, where dinner transforms into a victory for the resources. It's not just about central dishes; it's connected to night feasts featuring delightful stewed meats, scrumptious fish dishes, and authority pastas that raise your eating experience, making a gathering of flavors that dance on your taste buds.

➢ Sweet Endings Treat Pleasure:

No supper is done without a sweet conclusion. It's not just about the standard thing; It's about dessert happiness with corruptly rich chocolate cakes, fruity sorbets, and particularly prepared merchandise that wrap up your devouring involvement with a crescendo of charm, providing you with a persevering through impression of lavishness.

➢ Eating up for Merriment Remarkable Occasions:

Exceptional occasions demand remarkable eating encounters. It's not just about standard social events; it's connected to gobbling up for celebrations with spectacular platters of flavorful dishes, luxurious fish zeniths, and wanton multi-course eats that mark depictions of joy, joining friends and family in a superb eating experience.+

➢ Week's end Casual breakfast Brunching Party:

Finishes of the week are held for brunching party. It's not just about routine eats; it's about a week's end casual breakfast with mimosas, expert eggs Benedict, and various delightful cakes that change loosened mornings into culinary journeys of happiness.

➢ Outing Pleasures Outside Clean:

Nature allures with journey delights. It's not just about stuffed sandwiches; it's about outside style with epicurean cheddar sheets, charcuterie, and delectable finger food assortments that change picnics into classy culinary escapades under the open sky.

➢ Overall Gastronomy Worldwide Flavors:

Embrace the world on your plate with worldwide flavors. It's not just about regular dishes; It's about overall gastronomy with lively Thai curries, fragrant Indian biryanis, and great Italian lasagnas that license your taste buds to leave on a stormy culinary visit.

➢ Your Culinary Journey Starts:

This isn't just about meals; a culinary outing recognizes the range of tastes, the specialty of the show, and the enjoyment of sharing essential minutes around the table.

With these solid supper considerations for every occasion, you're ready to partake in the abundance of life through extraordinary eating, making each banquet a paramount occasion.

Welcome to the truth where your culinary choices aren't just about eating; they're connected to experiencing the wizardry of various and wonderful devouring.

Breakfast Recipes - Delectable Low-Carb Breakfast Thoughts for 2024

In the clamoring day break of 2024, the main feast of the day takes a cutting edge bend. It's not just about the typical breakfast; it's about a lively exhibit of low-carb breakfast thoughts that will entice your taste buds and launch your day on a sound note.

1. Avocado and Bacon Breakfast Bowl

Express welcome to a morning meal bowl that weds richness and firmness. It's not just about oats; it's about a bowl loaded up with ready avocados, firm bacon, poached eggs, and a sprinkle of hot sauce, making an orchestra of flavors that establishes the vibe for the afternoon.

2. Zucchini and Feta Egg Biscuits.

Hoist your morning meal with these egg biscuits. It's not just about the run of the mill biscuits; It's about exquisite zucchini and feta egg biscuits that are the ideal equilibrium between protein and flavor, making your morning a brilliant encounter.

3. Spinach and Mushroom Omelet Roll-Ups.

Omelets get a makeover with these roll-ups. It's not just about plain eggs; it's about an energetic blend of sautéed spinach, mushrooms, and feta cheddar moved up into a scrumptious bundle, making a morning work of art that is however gorgeous as it could be heavenly.

4. Smoked Salmon and Cream Cheddar Crepes.

Crepes don't have to be sweet illicit relationships. It's not just about sweet garnishes; It's about flimsy, sensitive crepes folded over smoked salmon, cream cheddar, escapades, and red onion, giving you a connoisseur breakfast that overflows with refinement..

5. Keto Chia Pudding with Berries.

Express farewell to sweet oats and embrace chia pudding. It's not just about oats; it's about a keto-accommodating chia pudding made with almond milk, chia seeds, and a variety of new berries, however nutritious as making a breakfast may be.

6. Greek Yogurt Parfait with Nuts and Berries

Parfaits are rethought for the low-carb period. It's not just about sweet granola; It's about Greek yogurt layered with toasted nuts, new berries, and a sprinkle of honey, giving you a delightful and outwardly engaging morning treat.

7. Green Smoothie Bowl.

Awaken to a bowl of energetic greens. It's not just about sweet oats; It's about a green smoothie bowl stacked with spinach, avocado, almond milk, and a sprinkle of seeds, carrying an invigorating and nutritious beginning to your day.

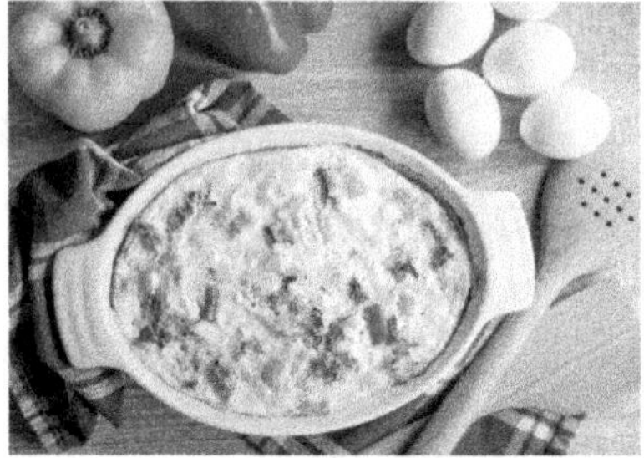

8. Yam and Hotdog Breakfast Skillet.

Skillets take on another personality with this generous breakfast. It's not just about plain potatoes; it's about a yam and frankfurter breakfast skillet with a vivid variety of veggies, eggs, and spices, making a one-dish wonder that fulfills your morning hunger.

➢ Your Morning meal Upset Starts:

2024 isn't simply one more year; it's a morning meal upset. With these low-carb breakfast thoughts, you're prepared to make your mornings heavenly, nutritious, and everything except standard.

Welcome to a reality where breakfast isn't just about daily practice; it's tied in with embracing the flavorful conceivable outcomes that every morning brings.

Lunch Recipes Supplement Stuffed and Advantageous Low-Carb Choices for 2024

Noon in 2024 is presently not about everyday sandwiches and convenient solutions. It's an amazing chance to fuel your body with supplement stuffed and helpful low-carb choices that fulfill your taste buds as well as keep you stimulated over the course of the day.

1. Barbecued Chicken and Vegetable Sticks:

Step into the universe of sticks where barbecued chicken blends with a rainbow of vegetables. It's not just about plain barbecued chicken; it's about a tasty blend of marinated chicken, chime peppers, zucchini, and cherry tomatoes strung onto sticks, making a lively, protein-rich lunch that is both fulfilling and outwardly engaging.

2. Cauliflower Rice Bowl with Tofu:

Embrace the low-carb insurgency with a cauliflower rice bowl. It's not just about conventional rice; it's about cauliflower rice sautéed flawlessly, finished off with marinated tofu, fresh vegetables, and a shower of sesame ginger sauce, making a helpful and carb-cognizant lunch that is however delightful as it could be healthy.

3. Mediterranean Quinoa Salad:

Mixed greens aren't only for calorie counters; they're for flavor lovers. It's not just about fundamental greens;

it's about a Mediterranean quinoa salad overflowing with variety and taste, highlighting quinoa, cucumbers, cherry tomatoes, kalamata olives, and feta cheddar, all prepared in a fiery lemon-oregano vinaigrette. This supplement stuffed choice will move your taste buds to the bright shores of the Mediterranean.

4. Portobello Mushroom Caprese Stack:

Give your lunch a connoisseur bend with a Portobello mushroom caprese stack. It's not just about customary sandwiches;

it's about enormous Portobello mushroom covers layered with ready tomatoes, new basil, mozzarella cheddar, and a shower of balsamic coating, making a low-carb show-stopper that is both filling and great.

5. Fish Avocado Lettuce Wraps:

Lunch in a hurry has never been this nutritious. It's not just about carb-loaded wraps; It's about fish salad settled in fresh lettuce leaves, with ready avocados and a smidgen of lime juice, making these wraps a helpful, low-carb choice that keeps you full and filled.

Dinner recipes flavorful and satisfying low-carb dinner choices

Supper Recipes: Delightful and Fulfilling Low-Carb Decisions for 2024 As the day slows down in 2024, supper is at this point not a dull everyday practice. It's a chance to enjoy delightful and fulfilling low-carb choices that tempt your taste buds, support your body, and set up for a serene night.

1. Lemon Garlic Spread Shrimp:

Hoist your supper with delicious shrimp washed in lemony garlic margarine. It's not just about plain protein; it's about stout, succulent shrimp sautéed in a lavish mix of garlic, lemon squeeze, and spread, making a dish that is wealthy in flavor and fulfillment.

2. Pesto Zoodles with Barbecued Chicken:

Bid goodbye to carb-weighty pasta and express welcome to zoodles. It's not just about standard noodles; It's about zucchini noodles covered in lively pesto and joined by barbecued chicken, cherry tomatoes, and a sprinkle of Parmesan cheddar, bringing a low-carb Italian magnum opus to your supper table.

3. Hot Wiener and Cauliflower Rice:

Prepare for supper with a kick. It's not just about plain cauliflower; it's about cauliflower rice sautéed with fiery wiener, chime peppers, and onions, making a generous and fulfilling low-carb choice that is loaded with flavor.

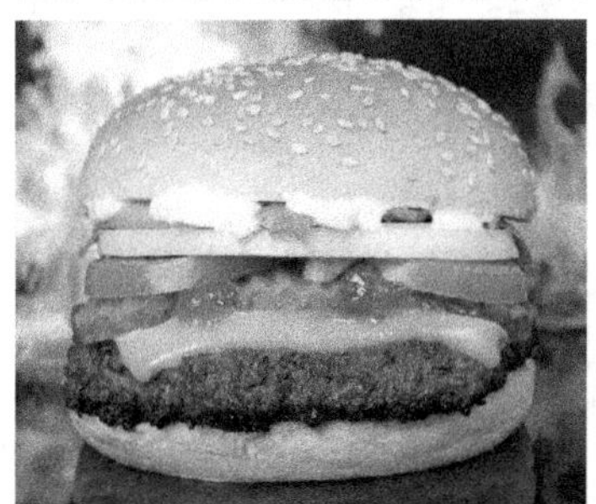

4. Hamburger and Broccoli Sautéed food:

Pan-sears are not generally held for takeout. It's not just about the oily eatery forms; It's about delicate cuts of hamburger, fresh broccoli florets, and an exquisite pan fried food sauce that you get ready at home, permitting you to partake in a low-carb supper that is however flavorful as it very well might be solid.

5. Stuffed Ringer Peppers with Ground Turkey:

Ringer peppers become vessels for a delightful supper, It's not just about tasteless stuffed peppers; it's about chime peppers loaded up with a combination of ground turkey, quinoa, dark beans, and flavors, finished off with liquefied cheddar and prepared flawlessly. This low-carb supper decision is a great contort on customary solace food.

6. Heated Lemon Spice Chicken:

Simmering an entire chicken isn't only for extraordinary events. It's not just about standard cooked chicken; it's about an entire chicken imbued with the kinds of lemon, garlic, and spices, making a succulent and fragrant magnum opus that is ideal for family meals or a weeknight treat.

7. Cauliflower and Spinach Lasagna:

Lasagna doesn't need to be carb-loaded. It's not just about pasta; It's about layers of cauliflower, spinach, ricotta, and mozzarella, prepared flawlessly in pureed tomatoes. This low-carb wind on an exemplary Italian most loved is both encouraging and nutritious.

➢ Your Supper Joy Starts:

Supper isn't simply one more dinner; it's a night charm that finishes your day. With these tasty and fulfilling low-carb supper choices, you're prepared to change your meals into culinary experiences that invigorate your taste buds and feed your body.

Welcome to the reality where supper isn't just about topping off; it's tied in with enjoying the rich prospects of tasty and fulfilling feasting.

Snack recipes are quick and healthy low-carb snacks

Nibble Recipes: Speedy and Solid Low-Carb Enjoyments for 2024 In the quick moving universe of 2024, snacks are presently not inseparable from culpability or split the difference. It's a period of fast and sound low-carb choices that conciliate your desires as well as keep your energy levels consistent over the course of the day.

1. Guacamole with Veggie Sticks:

Dunk into a universe of smooth goodness. It's not just about potato chips; it's about dynamic veggie sticks like cucumber, chime pepper, and carrot, matched with hand crafted guacamole that is wealthy in sound fats and flavor.

2. Cheddar and Nut Platter:

Guilty pleasure meets sustenance with a cheddar and nut platter. It's not just about sweet treats; it's about a determination of your number one cheeses, matched with blended nuts and a modest bunch of berries, offering a fantastic low-carb bite that is an orchestra of surfaces and tastes.

3. Greek Yogurt and Berries Parfait:

Fulfill your sweet tooth the sound way. It's not just about sweet treats; it's about Greek yogurt layered with new berries, a shower of honey, and a sprinkle of granola or nuts, giving you a bite that is both smooth and nutritious.

4. Smoked Salmon Cucumber Chomps:

Raise your eating with a dash of class. It's not just about oily chips; it's about daintily cut cucumber adjusts finished off with smoked salmon, a bit of cream cheddar, and a sprinkle of new dill. It is however refined as it seems to be great to make a tidbit.

5. Celery Sticks with Peanut Butter:

Rediscover the exemplary mix with a cutting edge turn. It's not just about sugar-loaded peanut butter cups; it's about crunchy celery sticks matched with all-normal nut or almond spread, offering a low-carb bite that is crunchy and fulfilling.

6. Avocado and Tomato Cuts with Olive Oil:

Avocado is the star of this basic yet fulfilling nibble. It's not just about customary chips; It's about avocado cuts showered with olive oil, sprinkled with ocean salt, and finished off with tomato adjusts, making a bite that is velvety, reviving, and wealthy in sound fats.

7. Hard-Bubbled Eggs with Mustard:

Eggs are a definitive protein-pressed nibble. It's not just about sweet energy bars; it's about hard-bubbled eggs prepared with a hint of mustard, offering a low-carb tidbit that is speedy to get ready and stacked with supplements

➢ Your Eating Unrest Starts:

2024 is your entryway to an eating upheaval. With these fast and solid low-carb choices, you're prepared to change your snacks into wonderful, nutritious minutes that keep your energy levels consistent and your taste buds enchanted. Welcome to the existence where tidbits aren't just about splitting the difference; they're about fast and sound guilty pleasures that supplement your bustling way of life.

Chapter 8

Sweetening the deal no sugar Ingredients and beyond

In our current reality where sugar has long held the high position as the dominant pleasantness supplier, 2024 is the year to reclassify the game. It's not just about the white precious stones; it's tied in with investigating the domain of no sugar fixings that convey pleasantness in a better, more regular, and frequently low-carb way.

1. Stevia: Nature's Sweet Leaf.

Express welcome to Stevia, nature's own sweet leaf. It's not just about refined sugar; it's about a plant-based sugar that comes from the Stevia rebaudiana plant, offering pleasantness without calories and carbs, making it a distinct advantage for those looking for a sugar substitute.

2. Priest Natural product: The Priest's Favoring.

Priest Organic product isn't your conventional natural product; the priest's favoring for those looking for pleasantness without the responsibility. It's not just about conventional sugar; it's about a characteristic sugar obtained from a priestly natural product that is heavenly, low-carb, and doesn't spike glucose levels.

3. Erythritol: The Sugar Liquor Darling.

Erythritol is the sugar liquor that adds to the arrangement. It's not just about customary sugar alcohols; it's about a characteristic sugar with an insignificant effect on glucose, settling on it a favored decision for those watching their carb consumption.

4. Xylitol: The Birch Excellence.

Xylitol isn't your typical sugar; it's the birch excellence of the sugar substitute world. It's not just about handled sugars; it's about a normally happening sugar found in birch trees and different plants that offers pleasantness without a similar effect on glucose.

5. Allulose: The Interesting Diamond.

Allulose is the uncommon jewel in the realm of sugars. It's not just considered normal sugars; a low-calorie sugar happens normally in little amounts in wheat, certain natural products, and, surprisingly, caramel, giving pleasantness without the responsibility.

6. Coconut Sugar: Nature's Sugar.

Coconut Sugar is nature's gift to the sweet-toothed. It's not just about table sugar; it's about a characteristic sugar obtained from the sap of coconut palm trees, offering a lower glycemic record and a remarkable caramel-like flavor.

7. Sans sugar Flavorings: The Key to Sweet Achievement.

Improve your culinary manifestations with sans sugar flavorings. It's not just about high-sugar extricates;

concentrates and flavorings are without sugar, permitting you to add profundity and pleasantness to your dishes without the extra carbs.

8. Regular Sugars A Better Way to Pleasantness:

The period of sugar has developed, and regular sugars have become the overwhelming focus. It's not just about void calories; it's tied in with embracing a better way to pleasantness with choices that are kinder to your body while still fulfilling your desires.

➤ Your Pleasantness Advancement Starts.

2024 imprints the sweet upheaval, where sugar's rule is tested by no sugar fixings and regular sugars that offer a better, low-carb, and flavorful way to pleasantness. Welcome to the reality where your pleasantness decisions aren't just about void calories; they're tied in with embracing a universe of no sugar fixings and options that improve upon the arrangement while remembering your wellbeing.

1. Finding Choices to Sugar for a Contemporary Low-Carb Way of life:

In the cutting edge scene of wellbeing cognizant living, the rule of conventional sugar is winding down, and choices are taking the spotlight. It's not just about the sweet gems; about finding a range of options, taking special care of contemporary low-carb ways of life, giving pleasantness without settling.

1. Priest Organic product: Nature's Gift to the Sweet Tooth

Express goodbye to refined sugar and welcome Priest Organic product, nature's gift to the sweet tooth. It's not just about the normal; it's about a characteristic sugar obtained from a priest organic product that conveys the commitment of delectable pleasantness without the responsibility, pursuing it as the ideal decision for low-carb lovers.

2. Stevia: The Natural Messenger of Pleasantness.

Stevia arises as the natural messenger of pleasantness, eclipsing the tradition of conventional sugar. It's not just about void calories; it's about a plant-based sugar obtained from Stevia rebaudiana that bestows a sweet flavor with zero calories and carbs, a momentous accomplishment for those chasing after a low-carb way of life.

3. Erythritol: The Sugar Liquor Whiz.

Enter Erythritol, the sugar liquor whiz that doesn't raise your carb count. It's not just about sugar alcohols; A normally happening sugar offers a similar pleasantness as sugar yet with negligible effect on glucose levels, a shelter for those embracing low-carb living.

4. Xylitol: Birch Tree's Sweet Confidential.

Xylitol is the sweet mystery that birch trees and different plants have imparted to the world. It's not just about normal sugars; about normally happening sugar's separated from birch trees and commits a normally sweet flavor without the cruel impacts on glucose.

5. Allulose: The Extraordinary Low-Calorie Sugar.

Allulose is the extraordinary low-calorie sugar that opposes the standards of sugar. It's not just about conventional sugars; low-calorie sugar happens normally in wheat, certain natural products, and, surprisingly, caramel, giving the pleasantness you need without undermining your low-carb way of life.

6. Coconut Sugar: Nature's Sense of Taste Pleaser.

Coconut Sugar arises as nature's sense of taste pleaser. It's not just considered normal table sugar; It's about a characteristic sugar extricated from the sap of coconut palm trees, offering a lower glycemic record and an unmistakable caramel-like flavor, settling on it the ideal decision for those embracing low-carb living.

7. Sans sugar Flavorings: The Unexpected, yet invaluable treasures.

Upgrade your culinary show-stoppers with sans sugar flavorings, the unexpected, yet invaluable treasures of your kitchen. It's not just about high-sugar separates; concentrates and flavorings are sans sugar, permitting you to add profundity and pleasantness to your dishes without agonizing over pointless carbs.

8. Normal Sugars: A Way to Better Extravagance.

In this contemporary low-carb period, the quest for pleasantness has advanced, and regular sugars have come to the very front. It's not just about sugar-loaded guilty pleasures; it's tied in with taking on a better way to fulfill your sweet desires with options that are kinder to your body while yet offering the sweet fulfillment you want.

Your Excursion to a Sweet Future Starts. 2024 is the beginning of a sweet insurgency where choices to sugar reclassify the contemporary low-carb way of life. Welcome to the existence where your sweet decisions aren't just about extravagance; they're tied in with finding a range of options that improve your life while adjusting impeccably with your well being cognizant objectives.

Crafting sweet treats without added sugar

In the period of careful living, the specialty of creating sweet treats has developed into an orchestra of flavors and wellbeing cognizant decisions. It's not just about sugar-loaded extravagances; it's about the imaginative excursion of making sweet treats without added sugars in 2024, changing pastry into a faultless pleasure.

1. Debauched Dim Chocolate Rapture

Enter the domain of debauched dim chocolate rapture, where the harshness of life's difficulties is improved by the lavishness of cocoa. It's not just about milk chocolate; it's tied in with picking great dim chocolate with a high cocoa content, bringing cell reinforcements and unadulterated, pure delight to your sense of taste.

2. Delicious Natural product Parfaits.

Organic product parfaits rethink pleasantness without the requirement for added sugars. It's not just about sweet organic product cups; it's tied in with layering ready natural products with Greek yogurt and a sprinkle of nuts or seeds, making a delectable pastry that is energetic, nutritious, and overflowing with regular pleasantness.

3. Nut Spread Joys.

Nut spread delights become the dominant focal point, offering an ensemble of surfaces and flavors. It's not just about sugar-loaded spreads; it's about unadulterated nut margarines that you can sprinkle over apple cuts or celery sticks, making a tidbit that is wealthy in solid fats and protein.

4. Healthy Heated Merchandise:

Heated merchandise is changed into healthy pleasures that catch the quintessence of regular pleasantness. It's not just about sweet biscuits and treats; recipes utilize ready bananas, unsweetened fruit purée, or dates to give the pleasantness and dampness, making them both nutritious and fulfilling.

5. Frozen Yogurt Pops:

Frozen yogurt pops carry cool reward with a sprinkle of pleasantness. It's not just about frozen yogurt; it's tied in with mixing Greek yogurt with normal natural product purees and freezing them into popsicles that extinguish your mid-year desires without added sugars.

6. Chia Seed Pudding:

Chia seed pudding is the embodiment of solid extravagance. It's not just about high-sugar puddings; it's about a smooth and nutritious pastry made by blending chia seeds with unsweetened almond milk or coconut milk, and letting the normal gelling properties of chia do something amazing.

7. Craftsman Cheddar Platters:

Craftsman cheddar platters reclassify dessert with complexity and energy. It's not just about sweet baked goods; it's about organized choices of fine cheeses, nuts, and dried natural products, conveying a sweet and exquisite experience that rises above customary sweet treats.

8. Sweet Spices and Flavors:

Open the capability of sweet spices and flavors to inject your dishes with regular pleasantness. It's not just about refined sugar; it's tied in with exploring different avenues regarding fixings like cinnamon, vanilla, and nutmeg to upgrade the normal kinds of your manifestations.

➢ Your Sweet Treat Transformation Starts:

In 2024, the specialty of making sweet treats without added sugars is an excursion of both culinary and wellbeing cognizant investigation. Welcome to a reality where your sweet guilty pleasures aren't just about void calories; they're tied in with creating magnum opuses that catch the pitch of normal pleasantness and rethink the manner in which you experience dessert.

Conclusion

Making Sweet Treats Without Added Sugars in 2024

In the period of careful living, the specialty of creating sweet treats has developed into an orchestra of flavors and wellbeing cognizant decisions. It's not just about sugar-loaded extravagances; it's about the imaginative excursion of making sweet treats without added sugars in 2024, changing pastry into a faultless pleasure.

1. Wonton Dim Chocolate Delight:

Enter the domain of wanton dim chocolate delight, where the sharpness of life's difficulties is improved by the extravagance of cocoa. It's not just about milk chocolate; it's tied in with picking excellent dim chocolate with a high cocoa content, bringing cell reinforcements and unadulterated, pure joy to your sense of taste.

2. Tasty Natural product Parfaits:

Organic product parfaits rethink pleasantness without the requirement for added sugars. It's not just about sweet organic product cups; it's tied in with layering ready natural products with Greek yogurt and a sprinkle of nuts or seeds, making a delectable pastry that is lively, nutritious, and overflowing with regular pleasantness.

3. Nut Spread Joys:

Nut spread delights become the dominant focal point, offering an orchestra of surfaces and flavors. It's not just about sugar-loaded spreads; it's about unadulterated nut margarines that you can sprinkle over apple cuts or celery sticks, making a tidbit that is wealthy in solid fats and protein.

4. Healthy Heated Merchandise:

Heated merchandise is changed into healthy pleasures that catch the substance of normal pleasantness. It's not just about sweet biscuits and treats; recipes utilize ready bananas, unsweetened fruit purée, or dates to give the pleasantness and dampness, making them both nutritious and fulfilling.

5. Frozen Yogurt Pops:

Frozen yogurt pops carry cool reward with a hint of pleasantness. It's not just about frozen yogurt; it's tied in with mixing Greek yogurt with regular natural product purees and freezing them into popsicles that

www.ingramcontent.com/pod-product-compliance
Lightning Source LLC
Chambersburg PA
CBHW070915260726
48661CB00004B/1737